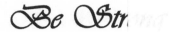

M000303143

The Holy Bible, NIV ©1984, Thomas Nelson, Inc.

KOBALT BOOKS

© Kobalt Books LLC
www.**kobaltbooks**.com

# Be Strong and Courageous

Be Strong and Courageous!
Do not be afraid or discouraged. For the Lord your God is
with you wherever you go. Joshua 1:9

# Be Strong and Courageous

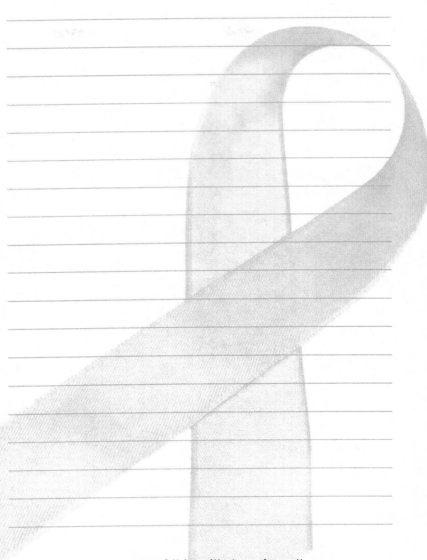

Jesus, aware of this, withdrew from there.
And many followed Him, and He healed them all.
Matthew 12:15

# Be Strong and Courageous

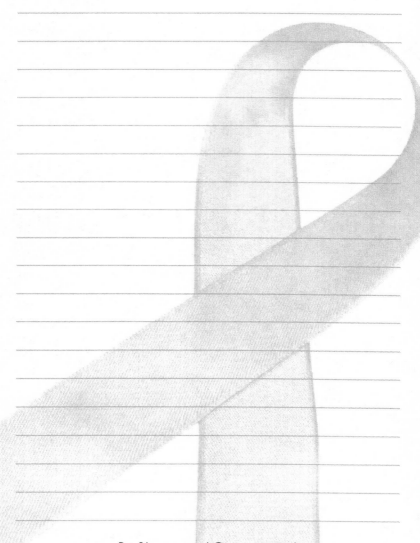

Be Strong and Courageous!
Do not be afraid or discouraged. For the Lord your God is
with you wherever you go. Joshua 1:9

# Be Strong and Courageous

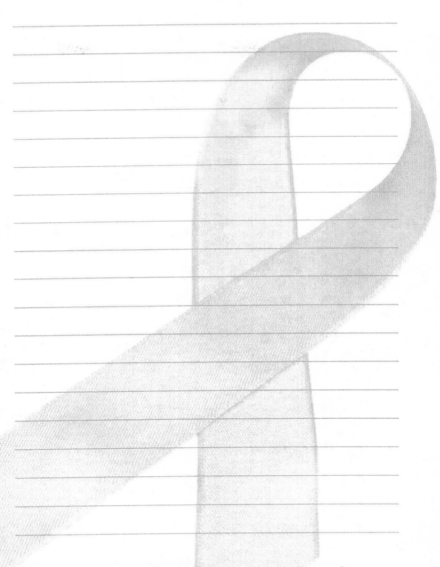

When He went ashore He saw a great crowd,
and He had compassion on them and healed their sick.
Matthew 14:14

# Be Strong and Courageous

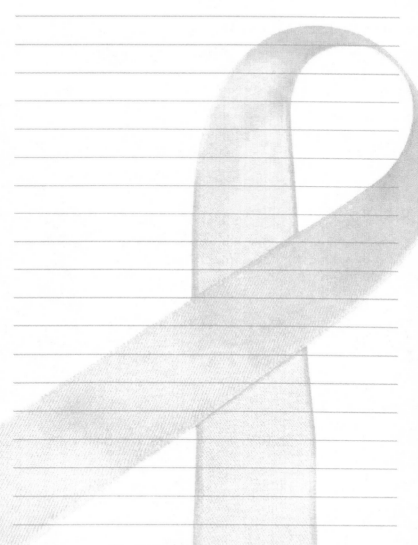

Be Strong and Courageous!
Do not be afraid or discouraged. For the Lord your God is
with you wherever you go. Joshua 1:9

# Be Strong and Courageous

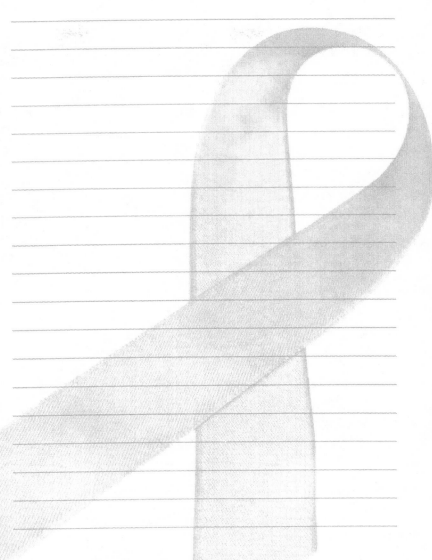

Seek the Lord and His strength;
seek His presence continually!
1 Chronicles 16:11

# Be Strong and Courageous

Be Strong and Courageous!
Do not be afraid or discouraged. For the Lord your God is
with you wherever you go. Joshua 1:9

# Be Strong and Courageous

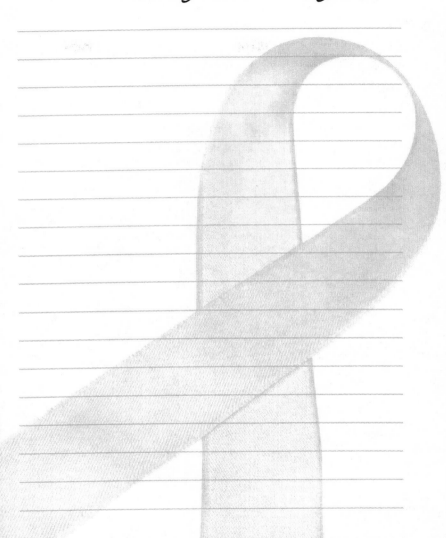

Be strong, and let us show ourselves courageous for the
sake of our people and for the cities of our God; and may
the Lord do what is good in His sight.
1 Chronicles 19:13

# Be Strong and Courageous

Be Strong and Courageous!
Do not be afraid or discouraged. For the Lord your God is
with you wherever you go. Joshua 1:9

# Be Strong and Courageous

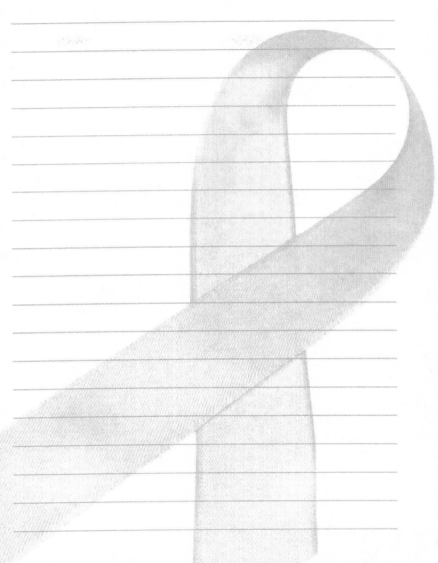

Be strong and courageous. Fear not; do not be dismayed.
1 Chronicles 22:13

# Be Strong and Courageous

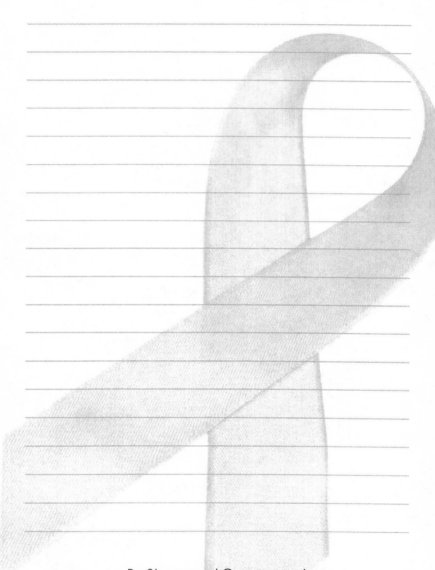

Be Strong and Courageous!
Do not be afraid or discouraged. For the Lord your God is
with you wherever you go. Joshua 1:9

# Be Strong and Courageous

Do not be afraid and do not be dismayed, for the Lord God, even my God, is with you. He will not leave you or forsake you, until all the work for the service of the house of the Lord is finished. 1 Chronicles 28:20

# Be Strong and Courageous

Be Strong and Courageous!
Do not be afraid or discouraged. For the Lord your God is
with you wherever you go. Joshua 1:9

# Be Strong and Courageous

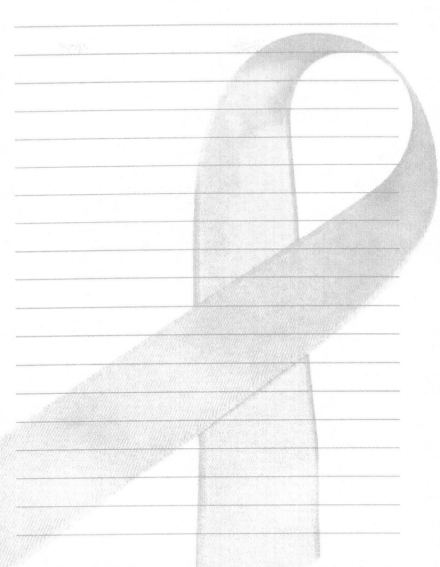

Be watchful, stand firm in the faith, act like men, be strong.
1 Corinthians 16:13

# Be Strong and Courageous

Be Strong and Courageous!
Do not be afraid or discouraged. For the Lord your God is
with you wherever you go. Joshua 1:9

# Be Strong and Courageous

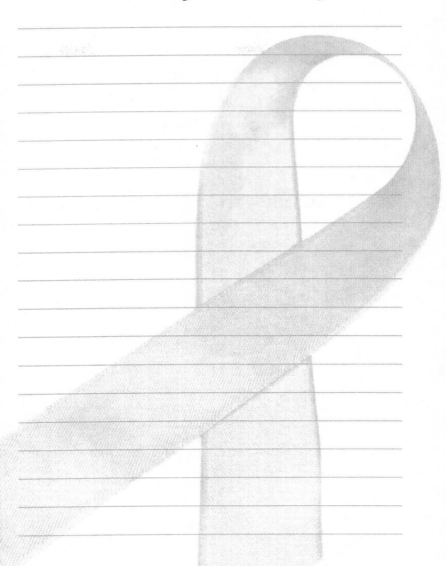

So you shall serve the Lord your God, and He will bless your
bread and your water. And I will take sickness
away from the midst of you. Exodus 23:25

# Be Strong and Courageous

Be Strong and Courageous!
Do not be afraid or discouraged. For the Lord your God is
with you wherever you go. Joshua 1:9

# Be Strong and Courageous

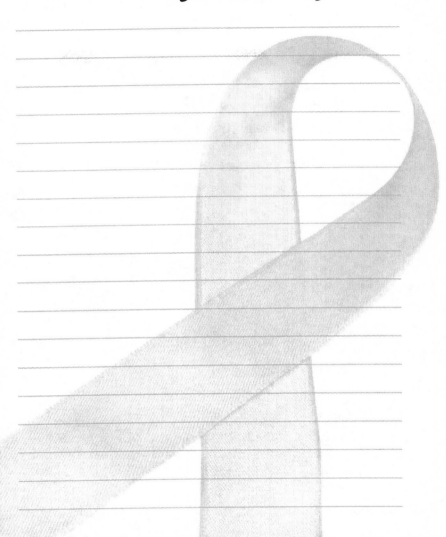

There is no fear in love; but perfect love casteth out fear:
because fear hath torment. He that feareth
is not made perfect in love.
1 John 4:18

# Be Strong and Courageous

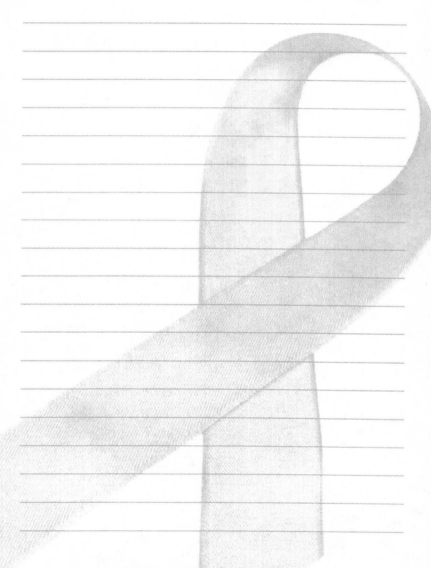

Be Strong and Courageous!
Do not be afraid or discouraged. For the Lord your God is
with you wherever you go. Joshua 1:9

# Be Strong and Courageous

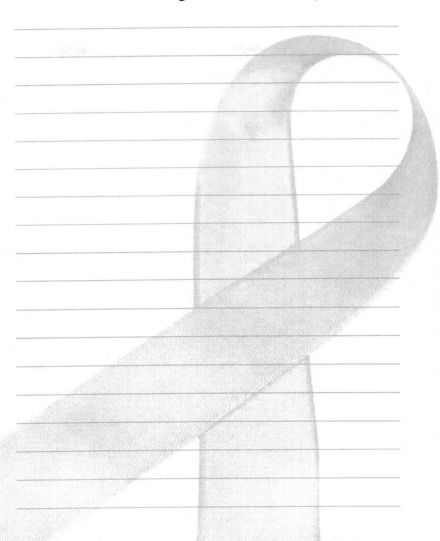

But sanctify the Lord God in your hearts: and be ready
always to give an answer to every man that asketh you a
reason of the hope that is in you with meekness and fear.
1 Peter 3:15

# Be Strong and Courageous

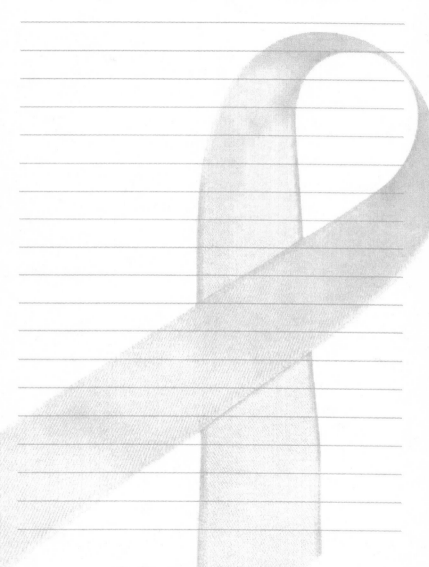

Be Strong and Courageous!
Do not be afraid or discouraged. For the Lord your God is
with you wherever you go. Joshua 1:9

# Be Strong and Courageous

And David said, The Lord who delivered me from the paw of the lion and from the paw of the bear, He will deliver me from the hand of this Philistine. And Saul said to David, Go, and may the Lord be with you. 1 Samuel 17:37

# Be Strong and Courageous

Be Strong and Courageous!
Do not be afraid or discouraged. For the Lord your God is
with you wherever you go. Joshua 1:9

# Be Strong and Courageous

Be strong and courageous, do not fear or be dismayed
because of the king of Assyria nor because of all the horde
that is with him; for the one with us is greater
than the one with him. 2 Chronicles 32:7

# Be Strong and Courageous

Be Strong and Courageous!
Do not be afraid or discouraged. For the Lord your God is
with you wherever you go. Joshua 1:9

# Be Strong and Courageous

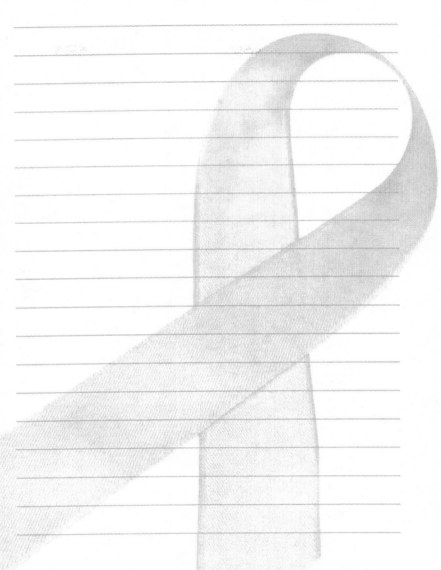

With him is an arm of flesh, but with us is the Lord our God,
to help us and to fight our battles.
2 Chronicles 32:8

# Be Strong and Courageous

Be Strong and Courageous!
Do not be afraid or discouraged. For the Lord your God is
with you wherever you go. Joshua 1:9

# Be Strong and Courageous

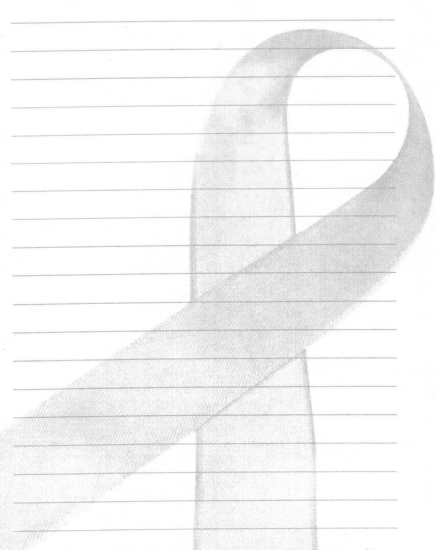

He delivered us from such a deadly peril, and He will
deliver us. On Him we have set our hope that
He will deliver us again.
2 Corinthians 1:10

# Be Strong and Courageous

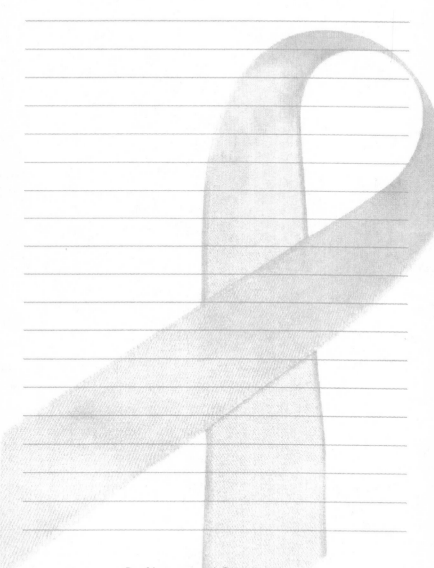

Be Strong and Courageous!
Do not be afraid or discouraged. For the Lord your God is
with you wherever you go. Joshua 1:9

# Be Strong and Courageous

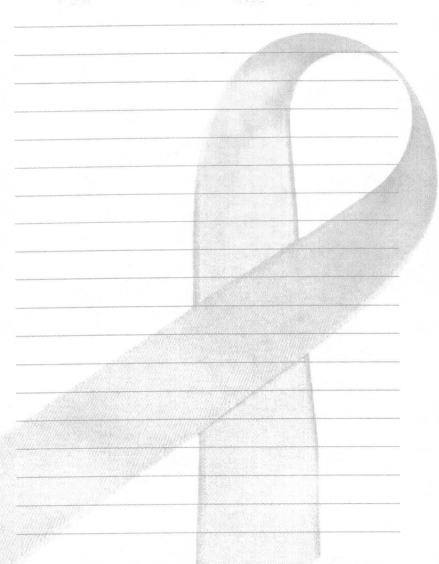

Indeed, we felt that we had received the sentence of
death. But that was to make us rely not on ourselves but on
God who raises the dead. 2 Corinthians 1:9

# Be Strong and Courageous

Be Strong and Courageous!
Do not be afraid or discouraged. For the Lord your God is
with you wherever you go. Joshua 1:9

# Be Strong and Courageous

Be strong, and let us show ourselves courageous for the sake of our people and for the cities of our God; and may the Lord do what is good in His sight. 2 Samuel 10:12

# Be Strong and Courageous

Be Strong and Courageous!
Do not be afraid or discouraged. For the Lord your God is
with you wherever you go. Joshua 1:9

# *Be Strong and Courageous*

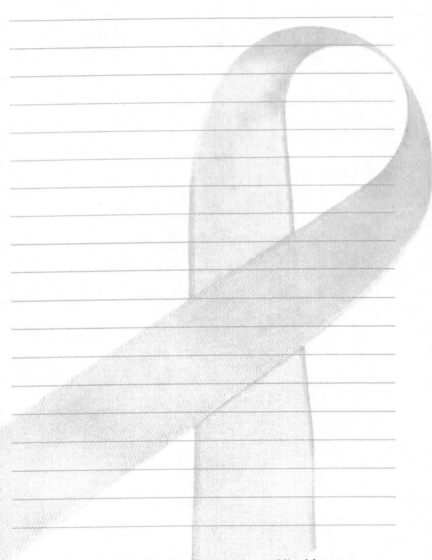

For God hath not given us the spirit of fear;
but of power, and of love, and of a sound mind.
2 Timothy 1:7

# Be Strong and Courageous

Be Strong and Courageous!
Do not be afraid or discouraged. For the Lord your God is
with you wherever you go. Joshua 1:9

# Be Strong and Courageous

By faith in the name of Jesus, this man whom you see and know was made strong. It is Jesus' name and the faith that comes through him that has completely healed him, as you can all see. Acts 3:12-26

# Be Strong and Courageous

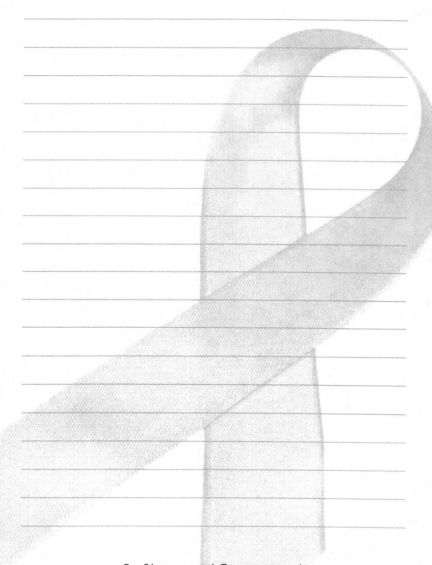

Be Strong and Courageous!
Do not be afraid or discouraged. For the Lord your God is
with you wherever you go. Joshua 1:9

# Be Strong and Courageous

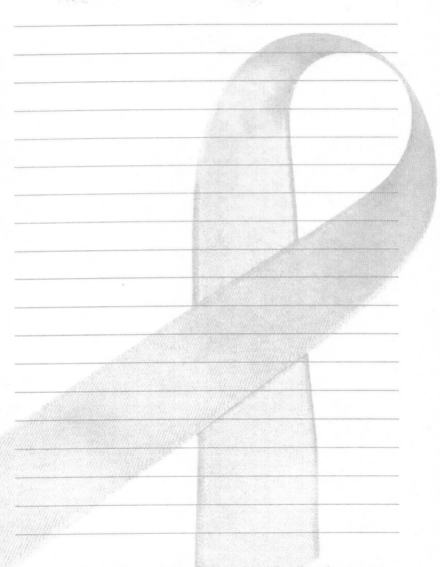

It is by the name of Jesus Christ of Nazareth, whom you crucified but whom God raised from the dead, that this man stands before you healed. Acts 4:10

# Be Strong and Courageous

Be Strong and Courageous!
Do not be afraid or discouraged. For the Lord your God is
with you wherever you go. Joshua 1:9

# Be Strong and Courageous

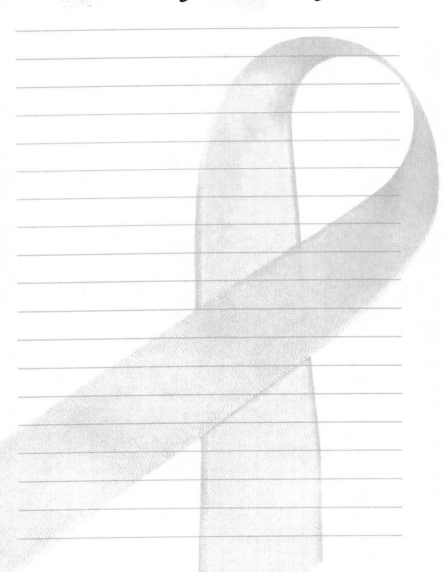

After they prayed, the place where they were meeting
was shaken. And they were all filled with the Holy Spirit
and spoke the word of God boldly. Acts 4:31

# Be Strong and Courageous

Be Strong and Courageous!
Do not be afraid or discouraged. For the Lord your God is
with you wherever you go. Joshua 1:9

# Be Strong and Courageous

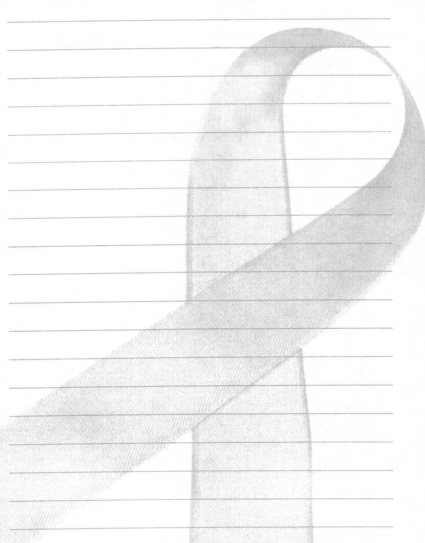

Be strong and courageous. Do not fear or be in dread of them, for it is the Lord your God who goes with you. He will not leave you or forsake you. Deuteronomy 31:6

# Be Strong and Courageous

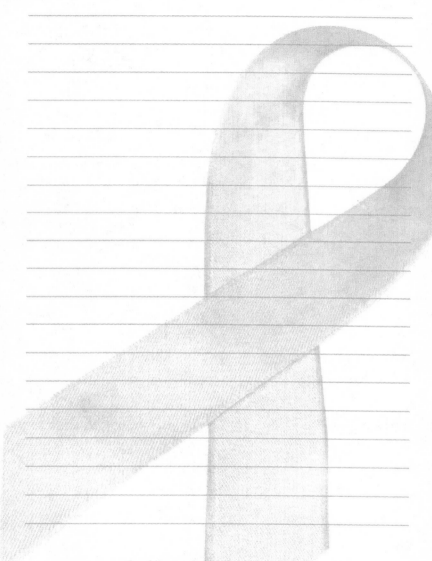

Be Strong and Courageous!
Do not be afraid or discouraged. For the Lord your God is
with you wherever you go. Joshua 1:9

# Be Strong and Courageous

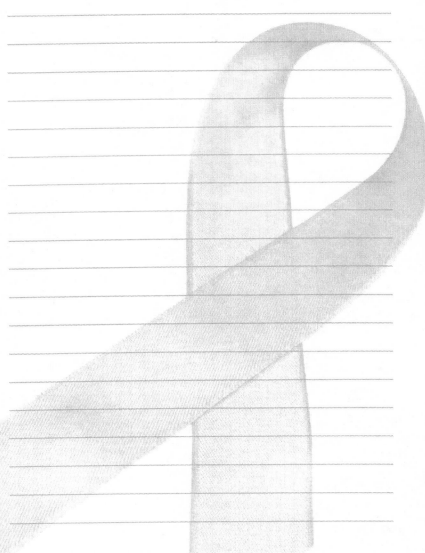

Finally, my brethren, be strong in the Lord,
and in the power of his might.
Ephesians 6:10

# Be Strong and Courageous

Be Strong and Courageous!
Do not be afraid or discouraged. For the Lord your God is
with you wherever you go. Joshua 1:9

# Be Strong and Courageous

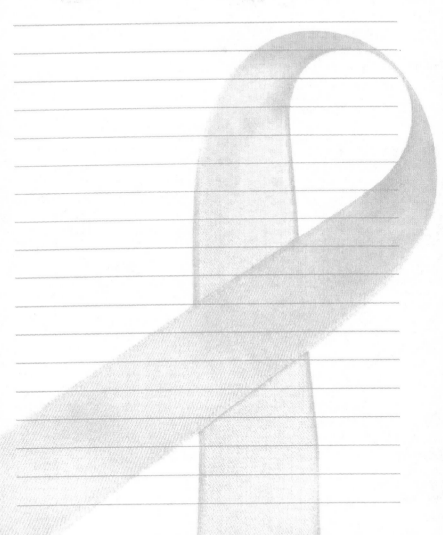

You shall serve the Lord your God,
and He will bless your bread and your water,
and I will take sickness away from among you.
Exodus 23:25

# Be Strong and Courageous

Be Strong and Courageous!
Do not be afraid or discouraged. For the Lord your God is
with you wherever you go. Joshua 1:9

# Be Strong and Courageous

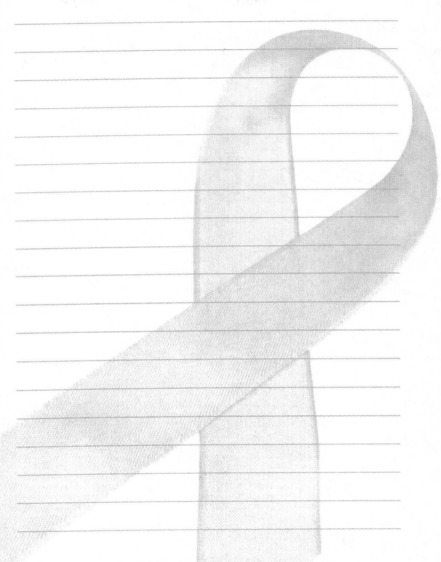

But for this purpose I have raised you up,
to show you my power, so that my name may be
proclaimed in all the earth. Exodus 9:16

# Be Strong and Courageous

Be Strong and Courageous!
Do not be afraid or discouraged. For the Lord your God is
with you wherever you go. Joshua 1:9

# Be Strong and Courageous

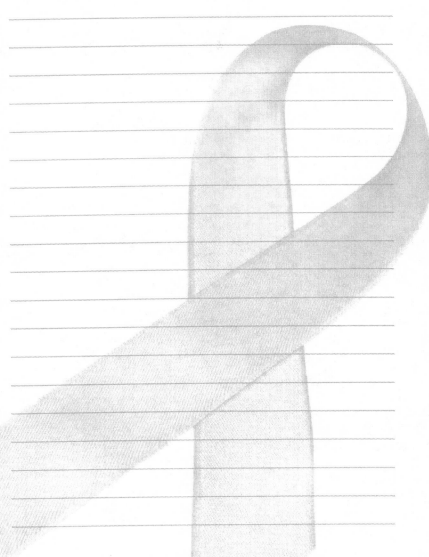

Arise! For this matter is your responsibility,
but we will be with you; be courageous and act.
Ezra 10:4

# *Be Strong and Courageous*

Be Strong and Courageous!
Do not be afraid or discouraged. For the Lord your God is
with you wherever you go. Joshua 1:9

# Be Strong and Courageous

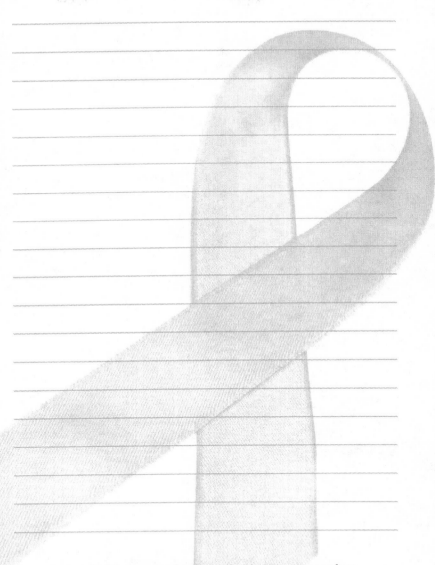

Let us hold unswervingly to the hope we profess,
for He who promised is faithful.
Hebrews 10:23

# Be Strong and Courageous

Be Strong and Courageous!
Do not be afraid or discouraged. For the Lord your God is
with you wherever you go. Joshua 1:9

# Be Strong and Courageous

Keep your life free from love of money, and be content
with what you have, for He has said,
I will never leave you nor forsake you.
Hebrews 13:5

# Be Strong and Courageous

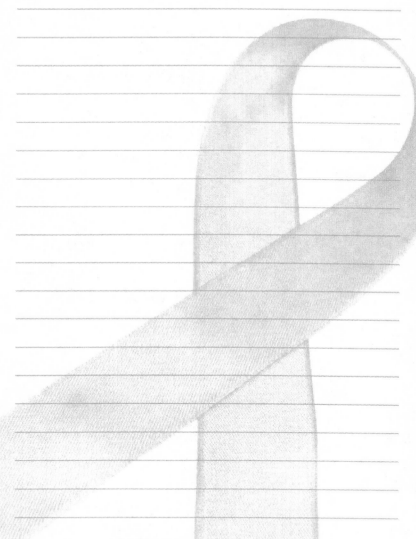

Be Strong and Courageous!
Do not be afraid or discouraged. For the Lord your God is
with you wherever you go. Joshua 1:9

# Be Strong and Courageous

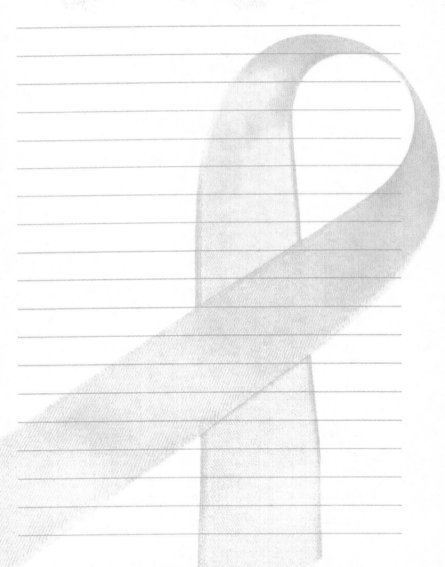

So that we may boldly say, The Lord is my helper,
and I will not fear what man shall do unto me.
Hebrews 13:6

# Be Strong and Courageous

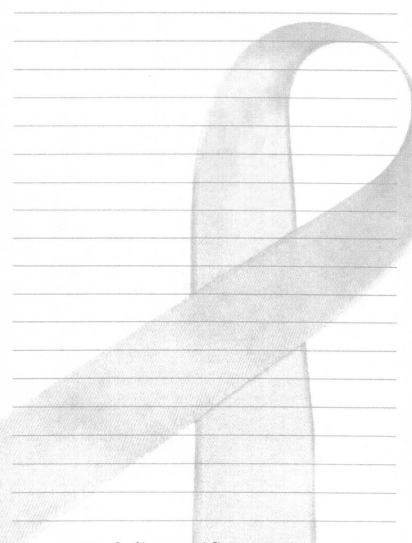

Be Strong and Courageous!
Do not be afraid or discouraged. For the Lord your God is
with you wherever you go. Joshua 1:9

# Be Strong and Courageous

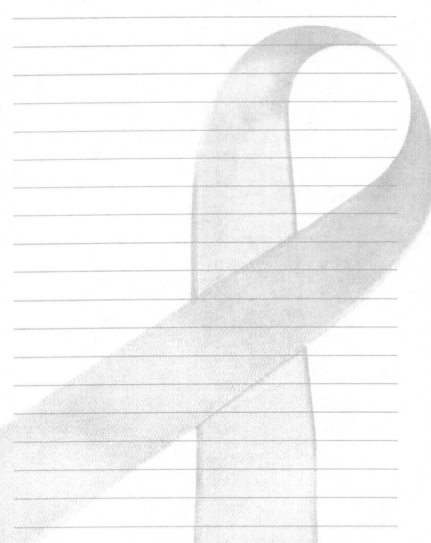

Therefore let us draw near with confidence to the throne of
grace, so that we may receive mercy and
find grace to help in time of need.
Hebrews 4:16

# Be Strong and Courageous

Be Strong and Courageous!
Do not be afraid or discouraged. For the Lord your God is
with you wherever you go. Joshua 1:9

# Be Strong and Courageous

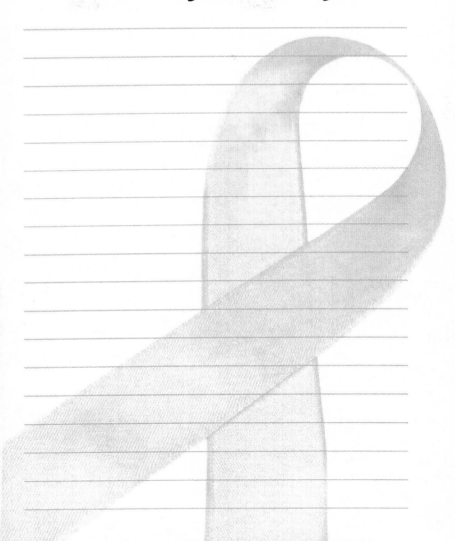

Behold, God is my salvation; I will trust, and will not be
afraid; for the Lord God is my strength and my song, and
He has become my salvation.
Isaiah 12:2

# Be Strong and Courageous

Be Strong and Courageous!
Do not be afraid or discouraged. For the Lord your God is
with you wherever you go. Joshua 1:9

# Be Strong and Courageous

Fear not, for I am with you; be not dismayed, for I am your
God; I will strengthen you, I will help you,
I will uphold you with my righteous right hand.
Isaiah 41:10

# Be Strong and Courageous

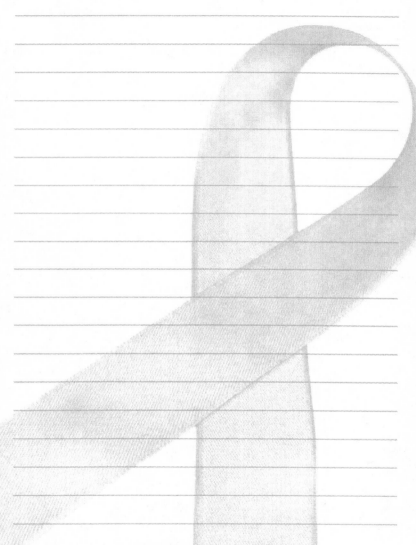

Be Strong and Courageous!
Do not be afraid or discouraged. For the Lord your God is
with you wherever you go. Joshua 1:9

# Be Strong and Courageous

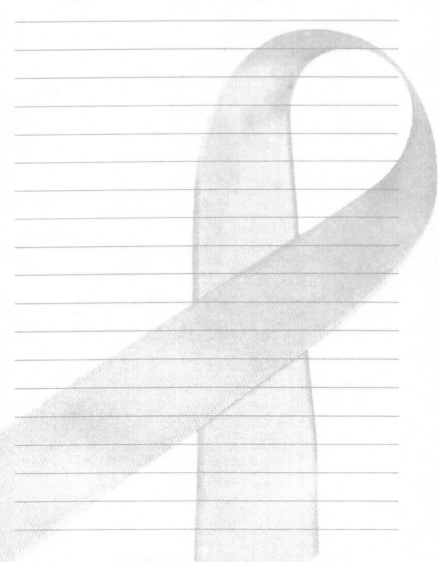

Each one helps his neighbor and says to his brother,
Be strong!
Isaiah 41:6

# Be Strong and Courageous

Be Strong and Courageous!
Do not be afraid or discouraged. For the Lord your God is
with you wherever you go. Joshua 1:9

# Be Strong and Courageous

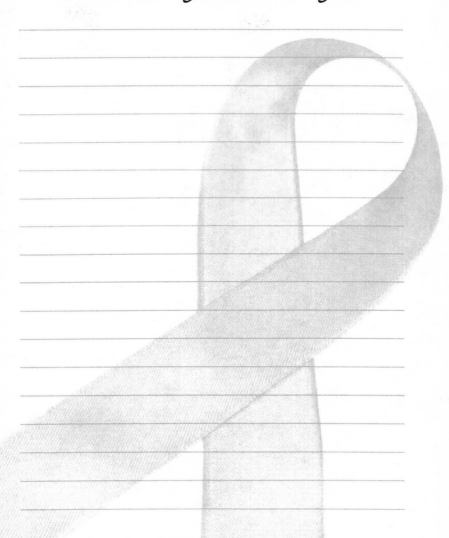

Then your light will break forth like the dawn, and your
healing will quickly appear; then your righteousness will go
before you, and the glory of the Lord
will be your rear guard. Isaiah 58:8

# Be Strong and Courageous

Be Strong and Courageous!
Do not be afraid or discouraged. For the Lord your God is
with you wherever you go. Joshua 1:9

# Be Strong and Courageous

You see that a person is justified by works
and not by faith alone.
James 2:24

# *Be Strong and Courageous*

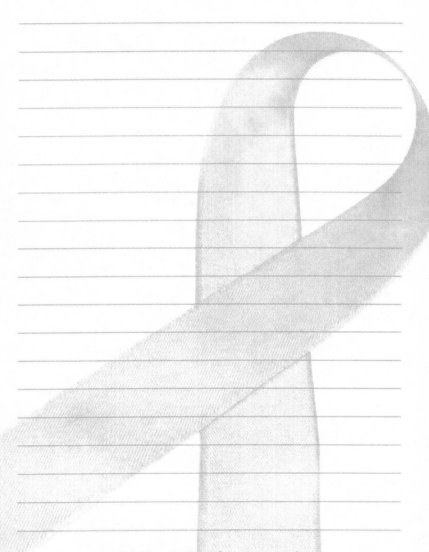

Be Strong and Courageous!
Do not be afraid or discouraged. For the Lord your God is
with you wherever you go. Joshua 1:9

# Be Strong and Courageous

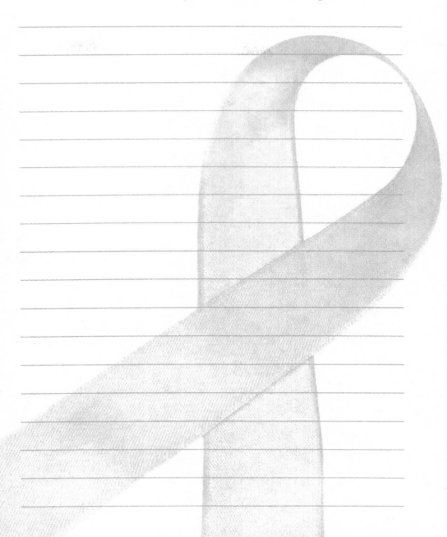

And the prayer of faith will save the one who is sick, and
the Lord will raise him up. And if he has
committed sins, he will be forgiven.
James 5:15

# Be Strong and Courageous

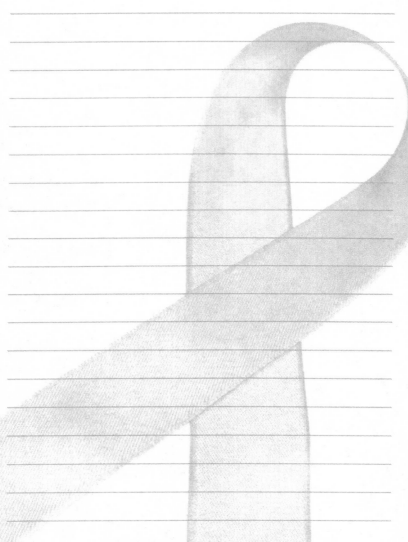

Be Strong and Courageous!
Do not be afraid or discouraged. For the Lord your God is
with you wherever you go. Joshua 1:9

# Be Strong and Courageous

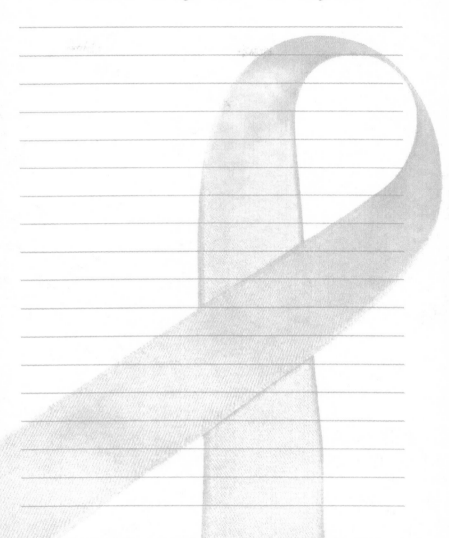

Therefore, confess your sins to one another and pray for
one another, that you may be healed. The prayer of a
righteous person has great power as it is working.
James 5:16

# Be Strong and Courageous

Be Strong and Courageous!
Do not be afraid or discouraged. For the Lord your God is
with you wherever you go. Joshua 1:9

# Be Strong and Courageous

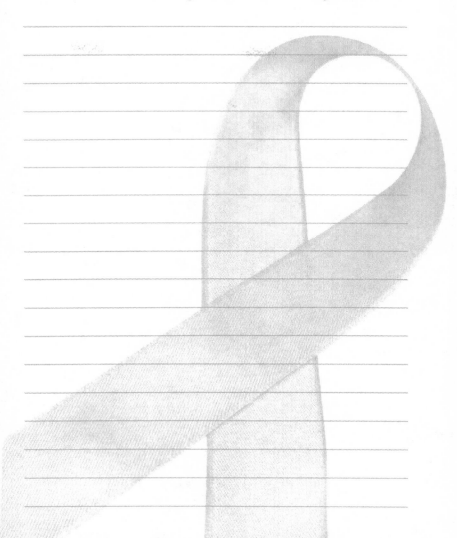

Heal me, O Lord, and I shall be healed;
Save me, and I shall be saved, For You are my praise.
Jeremiah 17:14

# Be Strong and Courageous

Be Strong and Courageous!
Do not be afraid or discouraged. For the Lord your God is
with you wherever you go. Joshua 1:9

# Be Strong and Courageous

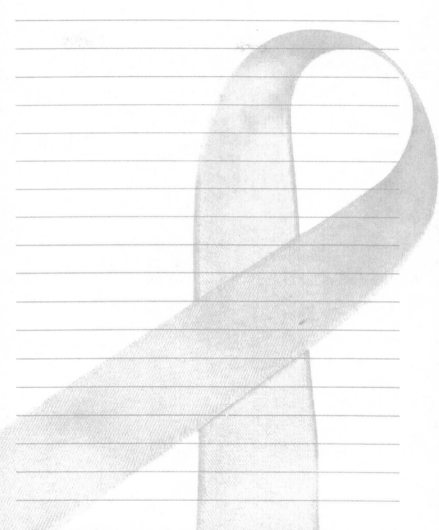

For I know the plans I have for you, declares the Lord, plans
for welfare and not for evil,
to give you a future and a hope.
Jeremiah 29:11

# Be Strong and Courageous

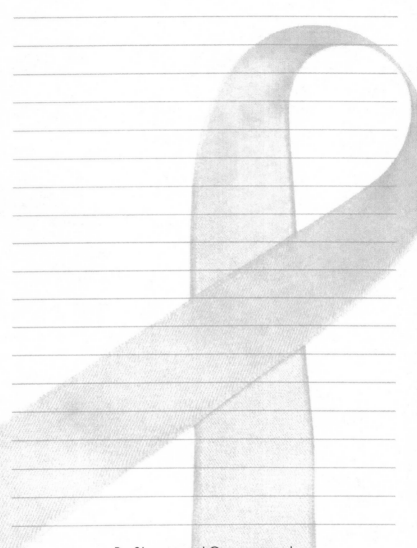

Be Strong and Courageous!
Do not be afraid or discouraged. For the Lord your God is
with you wherever you go. Joshua 1:9

# *Be Strong and Courageous*

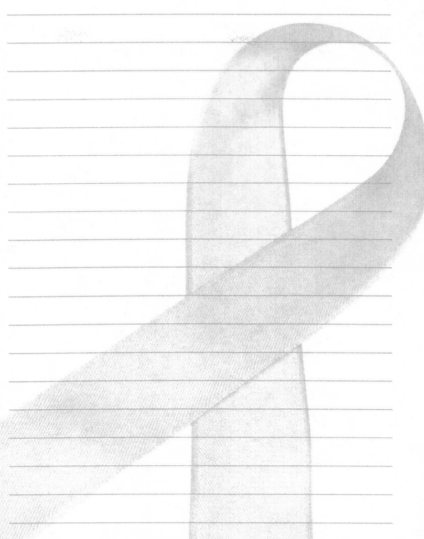

For I will restore health to you, and your wounds I will heal,
declares the Lord, because they have
called you an outcast. Jeremiah 30:17

# Be Strong and Courageous

Be Strong and Courageous!
Do not be afraid or discouraged. For the Lord your God is
with you wherever you go. Joshua 1:9

# Be Strong and Courageous

In Him was life, and the life was the light of men.
The light shines in the darkness,
and the darkness has not overcome it. John 1:4-5

# *Be Strong and Courageous*

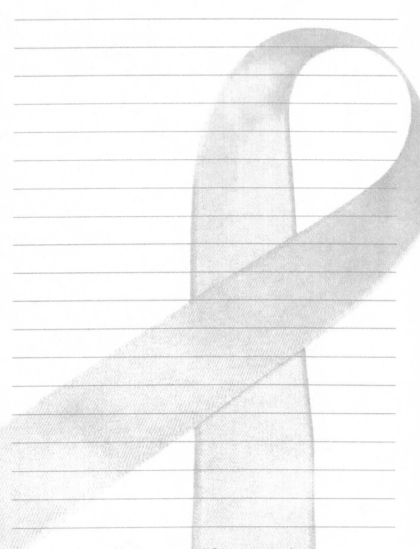

Be Strong and Courageous!
Do not be afraid or discouraged. For the Lord your God is
with you wherever you go. Joshua 1:9

# Be Strong and Courageous

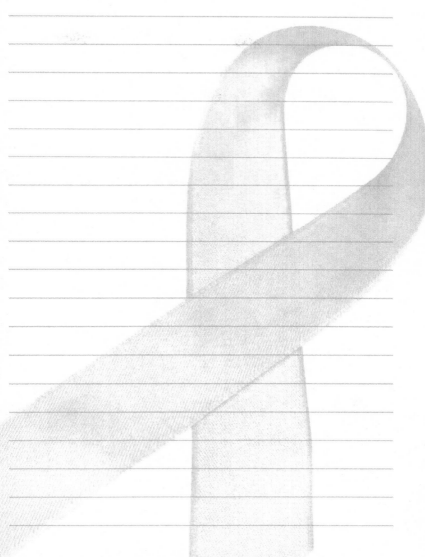

The thief does not come except to steal, and to kill, and to destroy. I have come that they may have life, and that they may have it more abundantly. John 10:10

# Be Strong and Courageous

Be Strong and Courageous!
Do not be afraid or discouraged. For the Lord your God is
with you wherever you go. Joshua 1:9

# Be Strong and Courageous

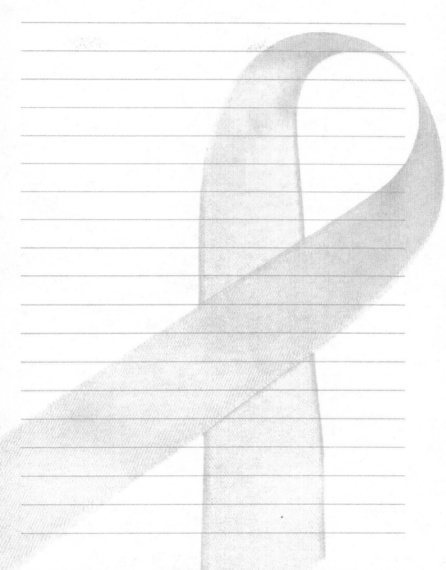

So they took away the stone. And Jesus lifted up his eyes
and said, "Father, I thank you that you have heard me."
John 11:41

# Be Strong and Courageous

Be Strong and Courageous!
Do not be afraid or discouraged. For the Lord your God is
with you wherever you go. Joshua 1:9

# Be Strong and Courageous

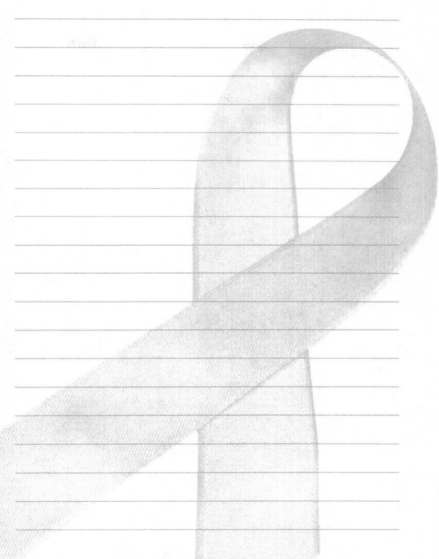

I knew that You always hear me, but I said this on account
of the people standing around, that they may
believe that You sent me. John 11:42

# Be Strong and Courageous

Be Strong and Courageous!
Do not be afraid or discouraged. For the Lord your God is
with you wherever you go. Joshua 1:9

# Be Strong and Courageous

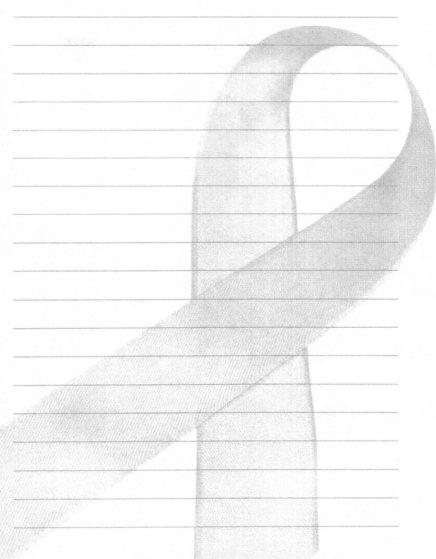

When He had said these things, He cried out
with a loud voice, "Lazarus, come out."
John 11:43

# Be Strong and Courageous

Be Strong and Courageous!
Do not be afraid or discouraged. For the Lord your God is
with you wherever you go. Joshua 1:9

# Be Strong and Courageous

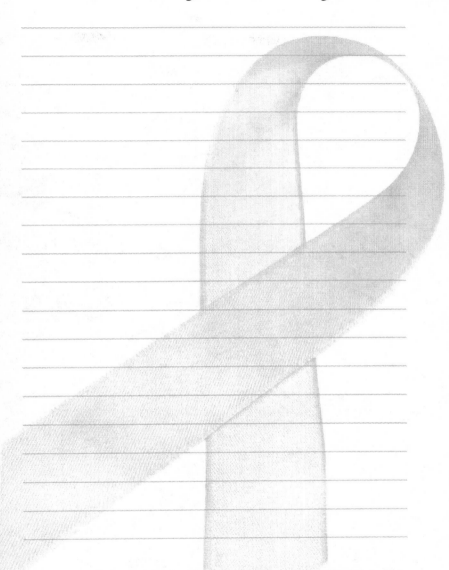

The man who had died came out, his hands and feet bound with linen strips, and his face wrapped with a cloth. Jesus said to them, "Unbind him, and let him go." John 11:44

# Be Strong and Courageous

Be Strong and Courageous!
Do not be afraid or discouraged. For the Lord your God is
with you wherever you go. Joshua 1:9

# Be Strong and Courageous

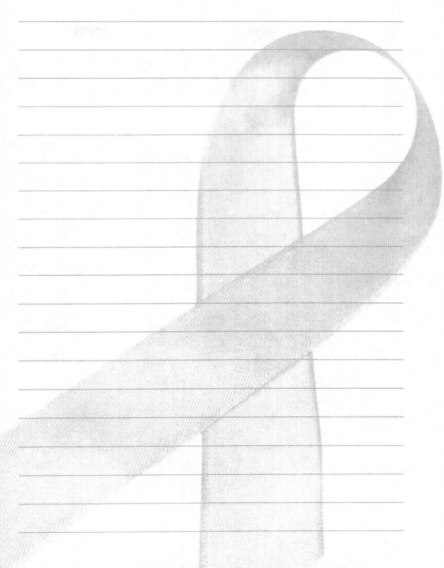

Many of the Jews therefore, who had come with Mary
and had seen what he did, believed in him.
John 11:45

# Be Strong and Courageous

Be Strong and Courageous!
Do not be afraid or discouraged. For the Lord your God is
with you wherever you go. Joshua 1:9

# Be Strong and Courageous

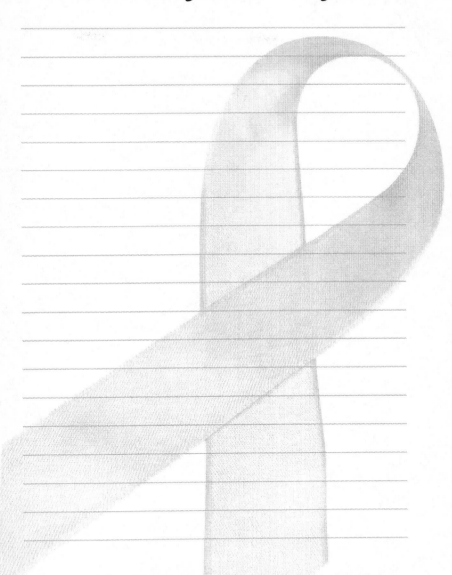

Peace I leave with you, my peace I give unto you: not as
the world giveth, give I unto you. Let not your heart be
troubled, neither let it be afraid. John 14:27

# Be Strong and Courageous

Be Strong and Courageous!
Do not be afraid or discouraged. For the Lord your God is
with you wherever you go. Joshua 1:9

# Be Strong and Courageous

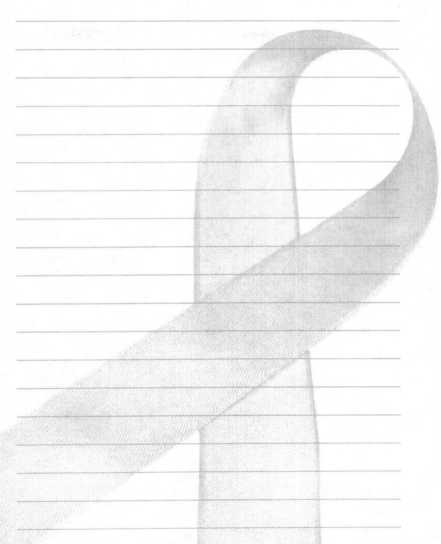

These things I have spoken unto you, that in me ye might
have peace. In the world ye shall have tribulation: but
be of good cheer; I have overcome the world.
John 16:33

# *Be Strong and Courageous*

Be Strong and Courageous!
Do not be afraid or discouraged. For the Lord your God is
with you wherever you go. Joshua 1:9

# Be Strong and Courageous

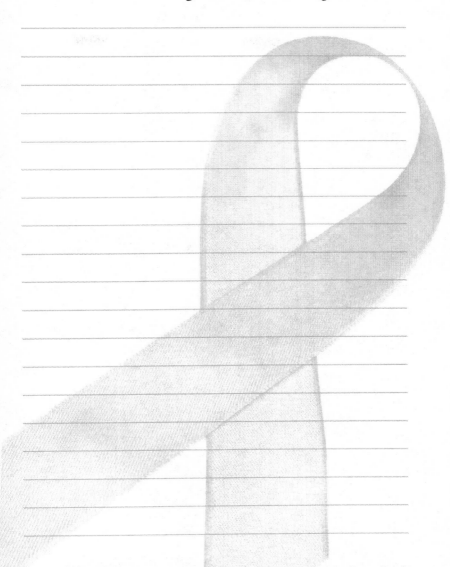

For God so loved the world, that he gave his only Son, that
whoever believes in him should not perish but
have eternal life. John 3:16

# Be Strong and Courageous

Be Strong and Courageous!
Do not be afraid or discouraged. For the Lord your God is
with you wherever you go. Joshua 1:9

# Be Strong and Courageous

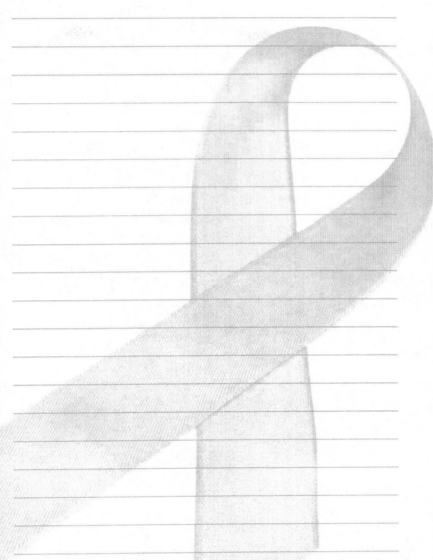

As soon as Jesus heard the word that was spoken,
he saith unto the ruler of the synagogue,
be not afraid, only believe. Mark 5:36

# Be Strong and Courageous

Be Strong and Courageous!
Do not be afraid or discouraged. For the Lord your God is
with you wherever you go. Joshua 1:9

# Be Strong and Courageous

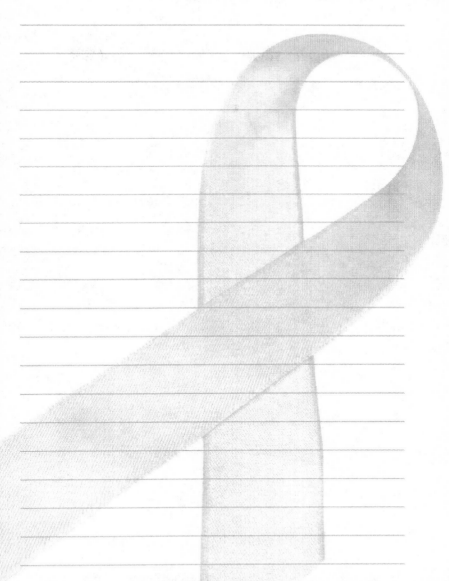

He said, Come. So Peter got out of the boat and walked
on the water and came to Jesus. Matthew 14:29

# Be Strong and Courageous

Be Strong and Courageous!
Do not be afraid or discouraged. For the Lord your God is
with you wherever you go. Joshua 1:9

# Be Strong and Courageous

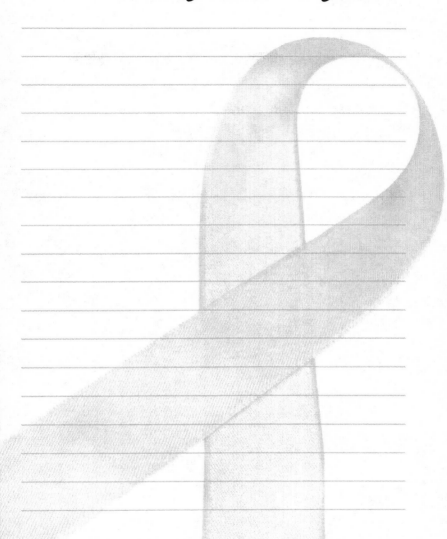

I eagerly expect and hope that I will in no way be
ashamed, but will have sufficient courage so that now as
always Christ will be exalted in my body, whether
by life or by death. Philippians 1:20

# Be Strong and Courageous

Be Strong and Courageous!
Do not be afraid or discouraged. For the Lord your God is
with you wherever you go. Joshua 1:9

# Be Strong and Courageous

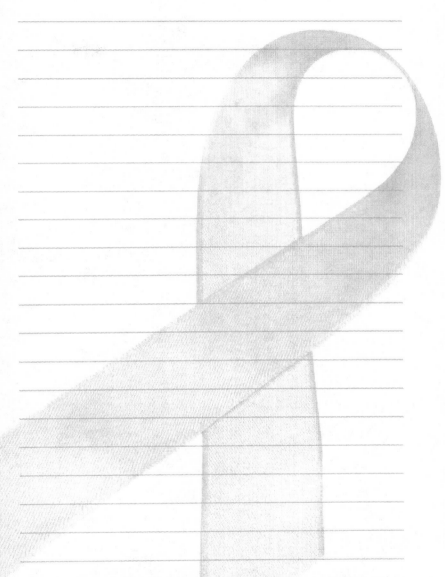

I can do all things through Christ which strengthens me.
Philippians 4:13

# Be Strong and Courageous

Be Strong and Courageous!
Do not be afraid or discouraged. For the Lord your God is
with you wherever you go. Joshua 1:9

# Be Strong and Courageous

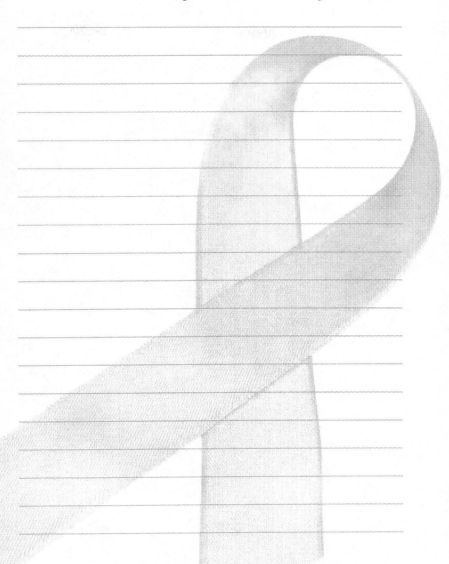

If you faint in the day of adversity, your strength is small.
Proverbs 24:10

# Be Strong and Courageous

Be Strong and Courageous!
Do not be afraid or discouraged. For the Lord your God is
with you wherever you go. Joshua 1:9

# Be Strong and Courageous

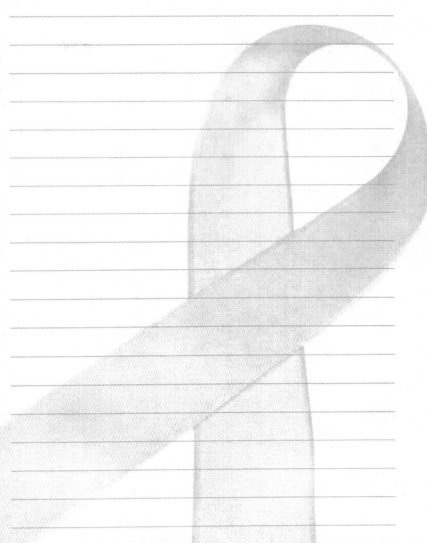

Trust in the Lord with all thine heart; and lean not unto thine
own understanding. In all thy ways acknowledge Him,
and He shall direct thy paths.
Proverbs 3:5-6

# Be Strong and Courageous

Be Strong and Courageous!
Do not be afraid or discouraged. For the Lord your God is
with you wherever you go. Joshua 1:9

# Be Strong and Courageous

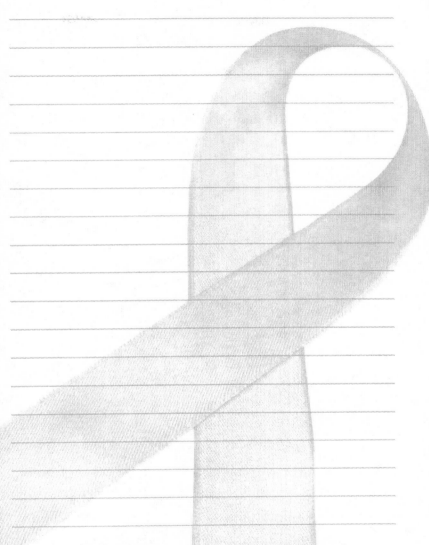

He sends forth His word and heals them and
rescues them from the pit and destruction.
Psalm 107:20

# Be Strong and Courageous

Be Strong and Courageous!
Do not be afraid or discouraged. For the Lord your God is
with you wherever you go. Joshua 1:9

# Be Strong and Courageous

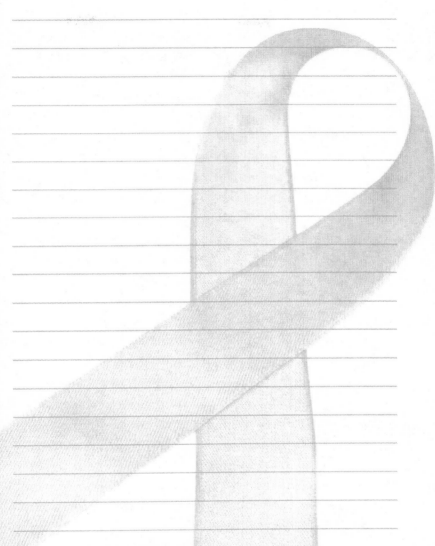

They will have no fear of bad news;
their hearts are steadfast, trusting in the Lord.
Psalm 112:7

# Be Strong and Courageous

Be Strong and Courageous!
Do not be afraid or discouraged. For the Lord your God is
with you wherever you go. Joshua 1:9

# *Be Strong and Courageous*

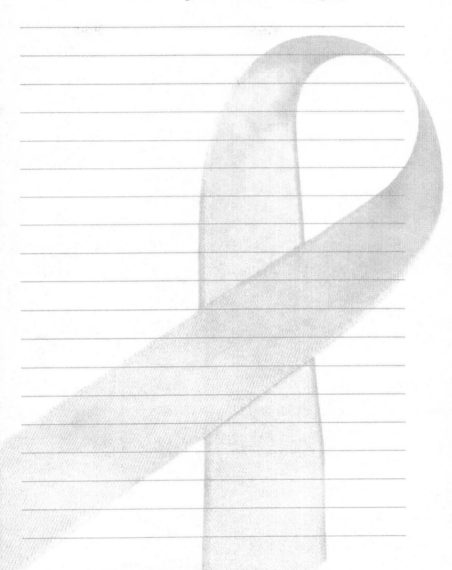

I have set the Lord always before me;
Because He is at my right hand, I shall not be shaken.
Psalm 16:8

# Be Strong and Courageous

Be Strong and Courageous!
Do not be afraid or discouraged. For the Lord your God is
with you wherever you go. Joshua 1:9

# Be Strong and Courageous

In my distress I called upon the Lord;
to my God I cried for help. From His temple
He heard my voice, and my cry to Him reached His ears.
Psalm 18:6

# Be Strong and Courageous

Be Strong and Courageous!
Do not be afraid or discouraged. For the Lord your God is
with you wherever you go. Joshua 1:9

# Be Strong and Courageous

Yea, though I walk through the valley of the shadow of
death, I will fear no evil: for thou art with me;
thy rod and thy staff they comfort me.
Psalm 23:4

# Be Strong and Courageous

Be Strong and Courageous!
Do not be afraid or discouraged. For the Lord your God is
with you wherever you go. Joshua 1:9

# *Be Strong and Courageous*

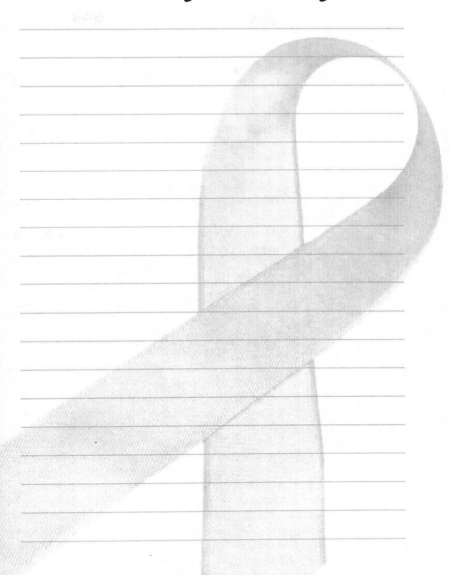

The Lord is my light and my salvation; whom shall I fear?
The Lord is the strength of my life; of whom shall I be afraid?
Psalm 27:1

# Be Strong and Courageous

Be Strong and Courageous!
Do not be afraid or discouraged. For the Lord your God is
with you wherever you go. Joshua 1:9

# Be Strong and Courageous

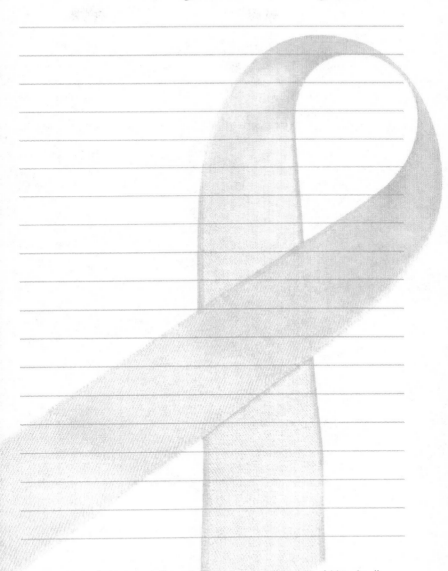

Wait on the Lord; Be of good courage, and He shall
strengthen thine heart; Wait, I say, on the Lord.
Psalm 27:14

# Be Strong and Courageous

Be Strong and Courageous!
Do not be afraid or discouraged. For the Lord your God is
with you wherever you go. Joshua 1:9

# Be Strong and Courageous

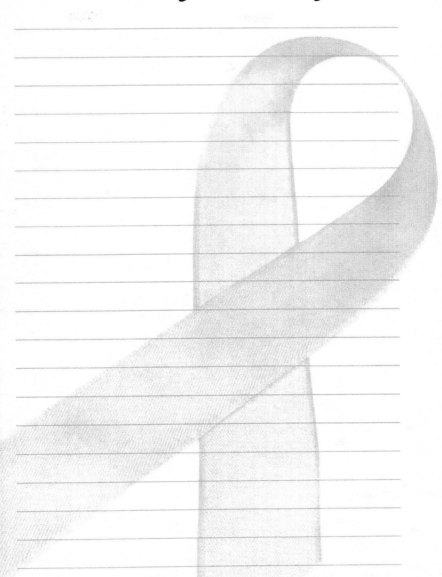

O Lord my God, I cried out to You, And You healed me.
Psalms 30:2

# Be Strong and Courageous

Be Strong and Courageous!
Do not be afraid or discouraged. For the Lord your God is
with you wherever you go. Joshua 1:9

# Be Strong and Courageous

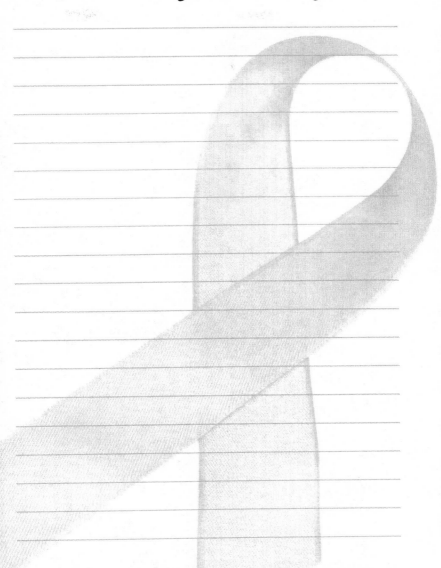

Be of good courage, and He shall strengthen your heart,
all ye that hope in the Lord.
Psalm 31:24

# Be Strong and Courageous

Be Strong and Courageous!
Do not be afraid or discouraged. For the Lord your God is
with you wherever you go. Joshua 1:9

# Be Strong and Courageous

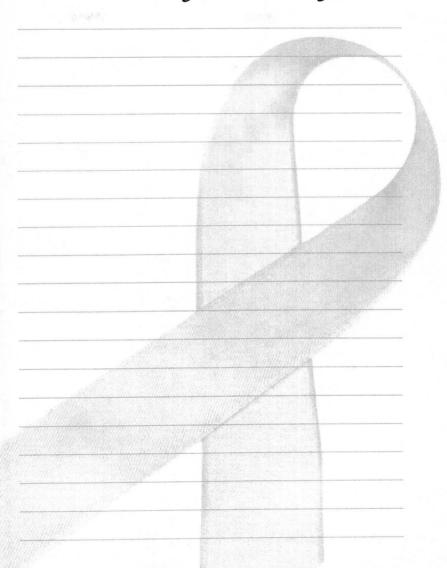

Our soul waits for the Lord; He is our help and our shield.
For our heart shall rejoice in Him, because we have
trusted in His holy name. Psalm 33:20-21

# Be Strong and Courageous

Be Strong and Courageous!
Do not be afraid or discouraged. For the Lord your God is
with you wherever you go. Joshua 1:9

# Be Strong and Courageous

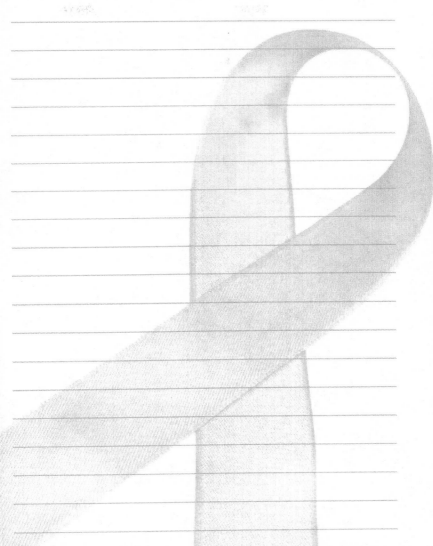

The eyes of the Lord are on the righteous, and his ears are
attentive to their cry; The righteous cry out, and the Lord
hears them; He delivers them from all their troubles.
Psalm 34:15,17

# Be Strong and Courageous

Be Strong and Courageous!
Do not be afraid or discouraged. For the Lord your God is
with you wherever you go. Joshua 1:9

# Be Strong and Courageous

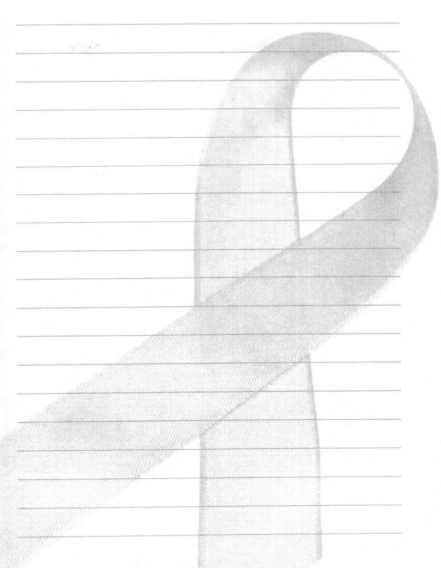

Many are the afflictions of the righteous,
but the Lord delivers him out of them all.
Psalms 34:19

# Be Strong and Courageous

Be Strong and Courageous!
Do not be afraid or discouraged. For the Lord your God is
with you wherever you go. Joshua 1:9

# Be Strong and Courageous

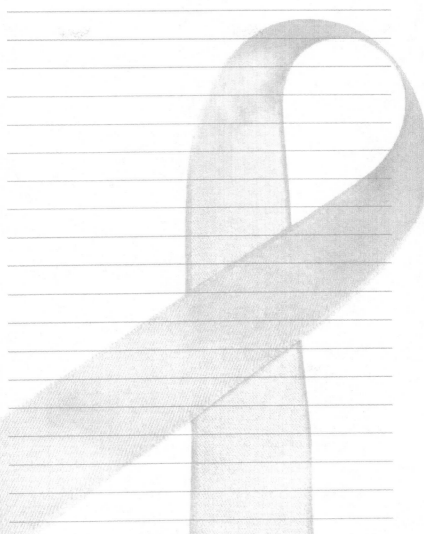

God is our refuge and strength,
a very present help in trouble.
Psalm 46:1

# Be Strong and Courageous

Be Strong and Courageous!
Do not be afraid or discouraged. For the Lord your God is
with you wherever you go. Joshua 1:9

# Be Strong and Courageous

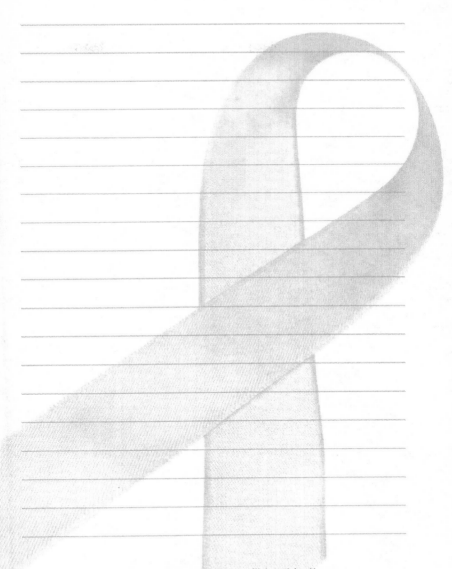

What time I am afraid, I will trust in thee.
In God I will praise his word, in God I have put my trust;
I will not fear what flesh can do unto me. Psalm 56:3-4

# Be Strong and Courageous

Be Strong and Courageous!
Do not be afraid or discouraged. For the Lord your God is
with you wherever you go. Joshua 1:9

# Be Strong and Courageous

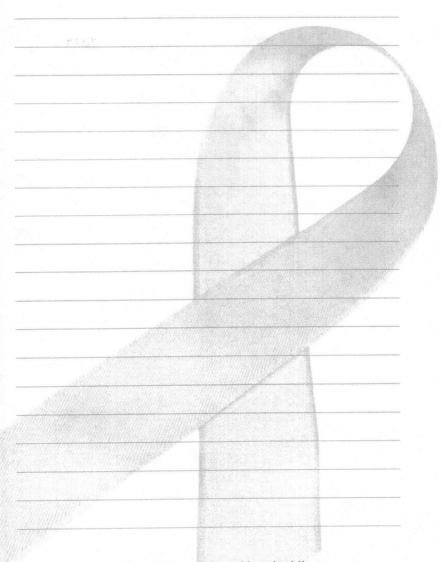

He sent out His word and healed them,
and delivered them from their destruction.
Psalms 107:20

# Be Strong and Courageous

Be Strong and Courageous!
Do not be afraid or discouraged. For the Lord your God is
with you wherever you go. Joshua 1:9

# Be Strong and Courageous

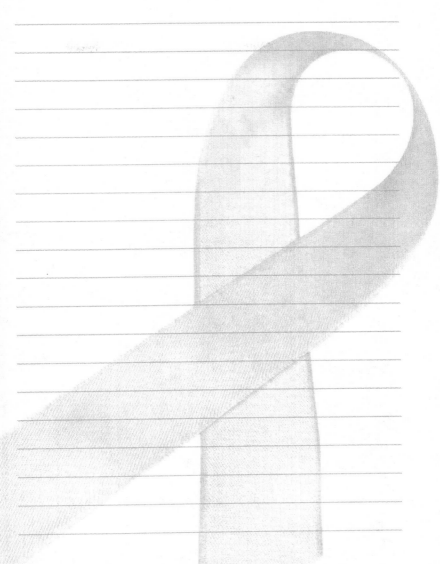

He shall not be afraid of evil tidings:
his heart is fixed, trusting in the Lord.
Psalms 112:7

# Be Strong and Courageous

Be Strong and Courageous!
Do not be afraid or discouraged. For the Lord your God is
with you wherever you go. Joshua 1:9

# Be Strong and Courageous

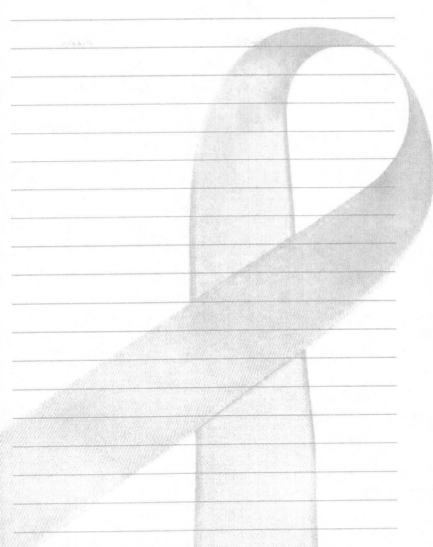

Wait on the Lord: be of good courage,
and He shall strengthen thine heart:
wait, I say, on the Lord.
Psalms 27:14

# Be Strong and Courageous

Be Strong and Courageous!
Do not be afraid or discouraged. For the Lord your God is
with you wherever you go. Joshua 1:9

# Be Strong and Courageous

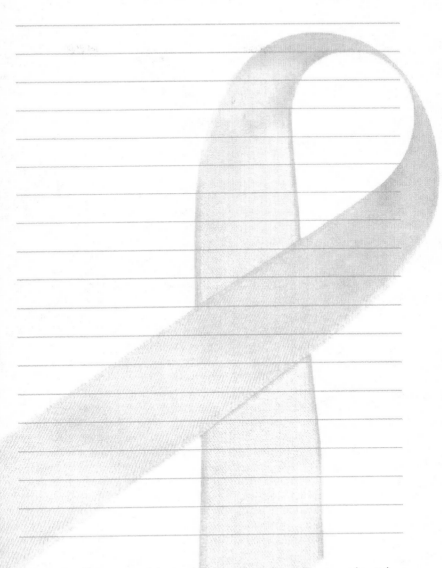

Be of good courage, and he shall strengthen your heart,
all ye that hope in the Lord.
Psalms 31:24

# Be Strong and Courageous

Be Strong and Courageous!
Do not be afraid or discouraged. For the Lord your God is
with you wherever you go. Joshua 1:9

# Be Strong and Courageous

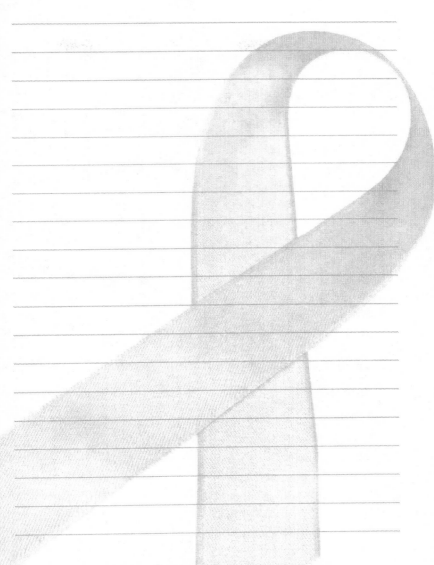

Many are the afflictions of the righteous,
but the Lord delivers him out of them all.
Psalms 34:19

# Be Strong and Courageous

_____

_____

_____

_____

_____

_____

_____

_____

_____

_____

_____

_____

_____

_____

_____

_____

_____

Be Strong and Courageous!
Do not be afraid or discouraged. For the Lord your God is
with you wherever you go. Joshua 1:9

# Be Strong and Courageous

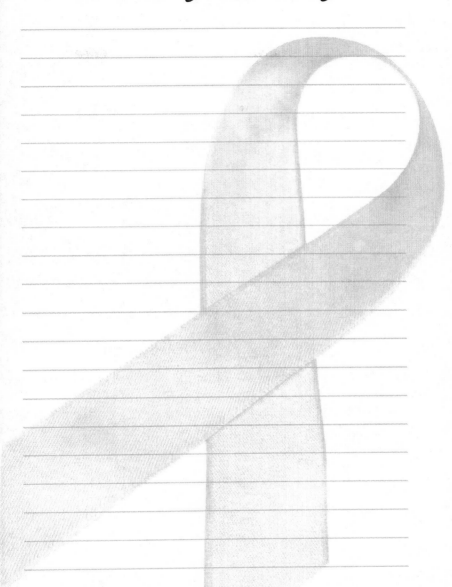

I shall not die, but live, and declare the works of the Lord.
Psalms 118:17

# Be Strong and Courageous

Be Strong and Courageous!
Do not be afraid or discouraged. For the Lord your God is
with you wherever you go. Joshua 1:9

# Be Strong and Courageous

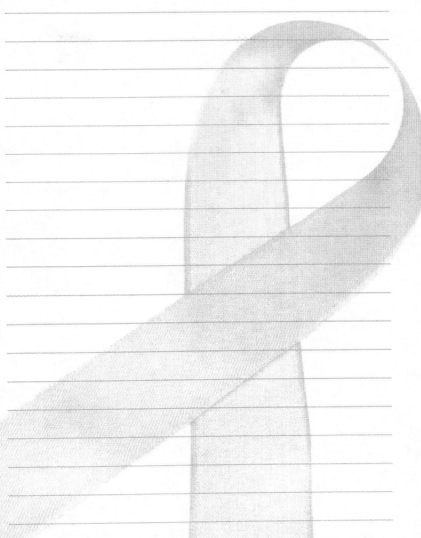

May the God of hope fill you with all joy and peace in
believing, so that by the power of the Holy Spirit
you may abound in hope.
Romans 15:13

# Be Strong and Courageous

Be Strong and Courageous!
Do not be afraid or discouraged. For the Lord your God is
with you wherever you go. Joshua 1:9

# Be Strong and Courageous

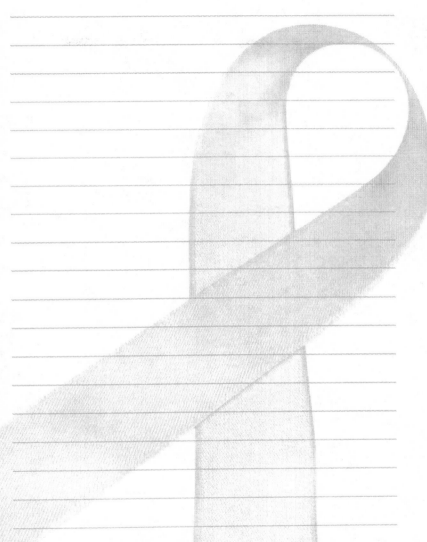

Not only so, but we also glory in our sufferings, because we
know that suffering produces perseverance;
perseverance, character; and character, hope.
Romans 5:3-4

# Be Strong and Courageous

Be Strong and Courageous!
Do not be afraid or discouraged. For the Lord your God is
with you wherever you go. Joshua 1:9

# Be Strong and Courageous

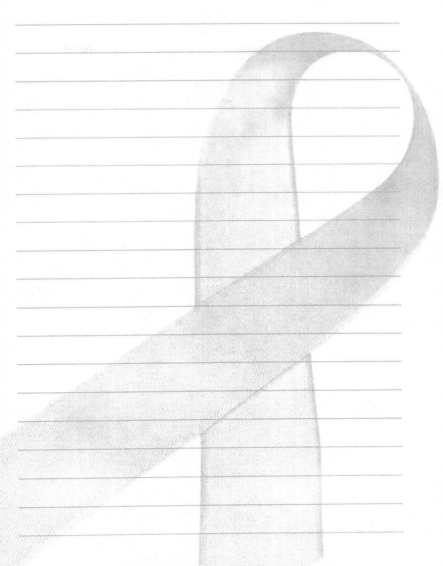

What then shall we say to these things?
If God is for us, who can be against us?
Romans 8:31

# Be Strong and Courageous

Be Strong and Courageous!
Do not be afraid or discouraged. For the Lord your God is
with you wherever you go. Joshua 1:9

# Be Strong and Courageous

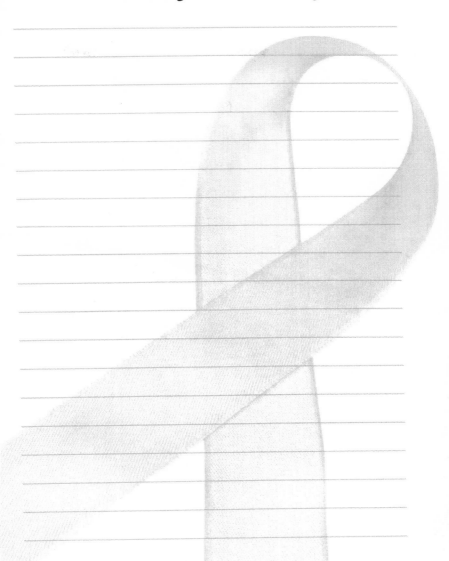

Yet in all these things we are more than
conquerors through Him who loved us.
Romans 8:37

# Be Strong and Courageous

Be Strong and Courageous!
Do not be afraid or discouraged. For the Lord your God is
with you wherever you go. Joshua 1:9

Made in the USA
San Bernardino, CA
16 October 2018